5
Tricks To Master
Diabetes, Both Type 1 & 2

Starter Kit and Guides to reinforcing insulin sensitivity, regulate high blood sugar, and lose weight| workouts and meal plans included

Lisa D. Mays

Disclaimer

This book is not intended to be a substitute for medical advice or treatment; any person with a condition requiring medical attention should consult a qualified medical practitioner or suitable therapist.

The information provided in this book is stated to be truthful and consistent, in that any liability, in terms of inattention or otherwise, by any usage or abuse of any policies, processes, or directions contained within is the

solitary and utter responsibility of the recipient reader. Under no circumstances will any legal responsibility or blame be held against the publisher for any reparation, damages, or monetary loss due to the information herein, either directly or indirectly.

Table of Content

WHO should try this book
Introduction

Chapter 1 The Disease-Diabetes

Different types of diabetes
Type 1 diabetes
Prediabetes
Type 2 Diabetes

Chapter 2 Mastering Diabetes Fundamentals

What Exactly Causes Insulin Resistance?
Can Insulin Be Revived?
Key Basics For Reinstalling Insulin Resistance
Weight Management

Disclaimer

This book is not intended to be a substitute for medical advice or treatment; any person with a condition requiring medical attention should consult a qualified medical practitioner or suitable therapist.

The information provided in this book is stated to be truthful and consistent, in that any liability, in terms of inattention or otherwise, by any usage or abuse of any policies, processes, or directions contained within is the

solitary and utter responsibility of the recipient reader. Under no circumstances will any legal responsibility or blame be held against the publisher for any reparation, damages, or monetary loss due to the information herein, either directly or indirectly.

Table of Content

WHO should try this book
Introduction

Chapter 1 The Disease-Diabetes

Different types of diabetes
Type 1 diabetes
Prediabetes
Type 2 Diabetes

Chapter 2 Mastering Diabetes Fundamentals

What Exactly Causes Insulin Resistance?
Can Insulin Be Revived?
Key Basics For Reinstalling Insulin Resistance
Weight Management

Chapter 3 Getting Started With Reversing Diabetes

Knowing Your Needs As A Diabetic
Food Guide

Trick 1 Starting A Healthy Low Gi Diet

How To Follow A Low GI Diet
Healthy Low GI foods
Sample Breakfast
Sample Lunch
Sample Dinner

Trick 2 Intermittent Fasting For Weight Loss And Reestablishing Insulin Sensitivity

Everything You Need To Know Before Getting Started With This Trick
How To Do It

Trick 3 Exercising To Regain Insulin Sensitivity

Why Do You Need To Exercise?
Suitable Exercise For Diabetics
5 Best Quick Exercise to keep you active

Trick 4 Knowing your pros and cons as a diabetic

10 Foods To Completely Avoid
10 Modification To Make Instead
Best Food List Diagram For Diabetes

Meal Plan & Recipes

Day 1
Breakfast: Berries & Walnut Crumble
Lunch: Red Pepper Dip served With Whole Grain
Vegetables
Dinner: Mussel and Crab Fry

Day 2
Breakfast: Ham & Cheddar Omelette
Lunch: Lentil Herbs Salad
Dinner: Peach Salmon
Day 3
Breakfast: Bread and Egg White with Oat
Lunch: Salsa Salmon Salad
Dinner: Quinoa Lime Beans Salad

Trick 5 Admiring Medical Necessity For Checkups

Who

Should Try This Book?

If you're a newly diagnosed person with diabetes. If your blood sugar rises beyond expectations everyday. If you once used to be an insulin dependent person but are currently experiencing too much low. If you've tried seeking out resources on the internet, or have even followed some medical instructions that still did not work for you. If you're a self determined person that keeps on doing the same thing over and over again, hoping to get better one day but it seems too capacitive and ineffective. If you feel desperate and hopeless about the disorder.

This book, 5 tricks to master diabetes, both type 1 and 2, has something you really need to know. From mistakes, causes, symptoms, down to remedies, including specified dieting and weight loss routines to aid your journey to battling diabetes.

Introduction

Diabetes has become one of the fast-rising chronic diseases currently booming in the United States and other parts of the World. It accounts for over 1.5 million fatalities annually according to the World Health Organization (WHO). When it comes to other leading causes of fatalities, diabetes is among the topmost, boosting the statistics to almost 20 million on yearly basis. Sounds tremendously scary.

Do you know that long term diabetes leads to;
Kidney disease
Heart attack
Hyperglycemia
Hypertension
Nerve damage
Retinopathy

Skin infections
Dental problems
Eye damages
Hearing impairment
Sexual dysfunction
Fungal cystitis
Stroke
Cancer
Dementia

Truth be told, diabetes can be scary, even life-threatening. But for picking up this book, it means that you're aware of the impairments caused by the disorder and you're indeed curiously ready to master it.

5 Tricks To Master Diabetes is more of a beginner's guide to help you keep going and prolong your happiness as a diabetic. It focuses on trying different scientifically proven and natural effective strategies to isolate the causes of diabetes and get rid of them. It's not another trend. It's a lifetime program. It encourages you to quit certain habits that worsens the disease, and recommends healthy, healing-worth ways to live instead.

Irrespective of the diabetes type you live with, the strategies in this book will provide you with naturally effective and motivating advice to prevent, manage, and even at some point reverse the disorder.

Key points you'll find in this book
Lose weight
Prevent progression
Proper dieting
Meal plans
Workouts
Reverse insulin resistance
Recover your full potentials
Thrive

Chapter 1

The Disease-Diabetes

Diabetes is a disease that determines when your blood sugar (glucose) is too high or subdued in control. It is an overweight condition no one can bear with ease. Diabetes in other words, is a conventional disorder that occurs when the functional organ in the body is unable to process insulin in the right order, or the pancreas is unable to provide insulin at all.

The pancreas is one of the most important organs in the human body that is positioned under the stomach and surrounded by the liver and small intestine. The pancreas helps the body function in two different ways; 1). an exocrine function that helps in digestion and 2). an endocrine function that regulates blood sugar. The endocrine component of the pancreas consists of islet cells (islets of Langerhans) that generate and release essential hormones directly into the bloodstream. Two of the main essential pancreatic hormones are 1). insulin, which operates to lower blood sugar, and 2). glucagon, which literally acts to elevate blood sugar.

To get it right, the absence of pancreas functions attracts insulin resistance. Persistent insulin resistance happens to cause diabetes. Insulin resistance is the cornerstar central culprit that evicts your chance for most chronic issues and undoubtedly the background for cardiovascular disease, type 2 diabetes, cancer, and obesity — all that province death. Unlike other causes, insulin resistance is one of the powerful forecasters of developing chronic disease in the meantime. According to one recent research, 65 percent of people living with type 1 diabetes for more than 20 years will die via cardiovascular disease and 50 percent of people living with type 1 diabetes for more than 30 years will die via kidney failure. However, managing or timing glucose to maintain blood sugar is not enough to secure you from diabetes complications in future. Insulin resistance doesn't uphold diabetes symptoms immediately. It takes approximately 20 years and luckily, it's detectable. And if you take essence to reverse insulin resistance today, you're paving the way for evicting several chronic conditions including diabetes in the future.

Different Types of Diabetes

There are so many reasons why your blood sugar may rise. The only way to exact the type of diabetes that you live with is through symptoms. Discover the difference between the most popular forms of diabetes below.

Type 1 diabetes

Type 1 diabetes is one of the main forms of diabetes that afflicts over 10 percent of the diabetes population. People refer to it as juvenile because it merely affects both young children and adolescents. It happens in reflection of an autoimmune strike that kills pancreatic islet cells (the insulin-producing organs). As a result of the autoimmune reflection, the body's self-made (*endogenous*) insulin production is decreased causing the body to crave for *exogenous insulin* (insulin injected via a pen, insulin pump, or spring). In some cases, metabolic syndrome are linked to factors triggering the autoimmune reflection which includes being exposed to stress and viruses, drinking or feeding infants with cow milk, and merely all inherited through genetic predisposition

When the insulin production organs become dysfunctional and die off in your body, your cells will be unable to make use of free-circulative glucose that accumulates in your bloodstream. At this time, glucose which is used as fuel for immune functionalities to work becomes complicated while the body would be left with the option to focus on fat stores for energy.

Energy subtracted from fat burn does not just leave the body in a normal state but makes the blood more acidic. The condition it results to is called diabetes ketoacidosis. Both long-term and short-term implications result as ketoacidosis progresses.

During this time, your body struggles and tries to unleash excess blood through the kidneys. That's when symptoms like steadily feeling thirsty and excessively peeing become part of a type 1 diabetes sufferer. Steady hunger while shading unnecessary weight follows up as time goes on. It will gradually become more and more unbearable and can invite death implication after so much unbearable pressure.

Restoration of the insulin in this case is possible but might alter due to some restrictions that must be followed. When suffering from T1D, there are possibilities according to several studies that you can live long for years if you eat a balanced, healthy diet and instructionally maintain the prescribed insulin availability whether through injections or pumps.

This approach works but is not enough for regaining insulin stability alone. That's merely because T1D mostly endorses sufferers with glycemic roller coasters, making them prone to several related complications.

Prediabetes

Prediabetes is a hardly detectable condition that precedes type 2 diabetes. Prediabetes occurs when your liver and muscles become invulnerable to normal insulin supply, causing a slight abnormality between glucose and insulin retention.

This occurrence allows glucose to invade your bloodstream which will elevate your fasting blood glucose (sugar).

Think of prediabetes as a significant sign that type 2 diabetes is right behind the corner. Prediabetes is usually diagnosed when fasting blood glucose is between 100-125 mg/dL, and sometimes, when your A1c is crossing between 5.7%-6.4% as elaborated in one study. Approaching the 5 tricks together in this condition will completely terminate insulin resistance and eliminate the fear of developing type 2 diabetes.

Type 2 Diabetes

Type 2 diabetes is the most popular form of the disorder that covers the population with over 90 percent diagnosed persons. They are of two forms which are 1). insulin-dependent that genetically occurs when prediabetic, fasting blood glucose exceeds 125 mg/dL, or when your A1c level is greater than 6.5 and you're no longer capable of manufacturing adequate endogenous insulins. And 2). non insulin-independent that excels when the prediabetic, fasting blood glucose exceeds 125 mg/dL, or when your A1c level is greater than 6.5, but you're still manufacturing adequate endogenous insulin.

Most people with type 2 diabetes suffer from metabolism syndrome (an ideology that represents the process that causes insulin resistance and also the circumstance whereby the insulin is completely ineligible to produce beta cells. Metabolic syndrome is related to the following risk factors;

- Excessive weight gain and belly fat
- High blood sugar and high blood pressure
- Diet rejection most especially carbs
- Genetics inheritance

T2D's most dangerous, yet overlooked risk factor is weight gain which can be detected in almost 80% out of 90% of people with type 2 diabetes.

Being obese or overweight increases the chance of type 2 diabetes by 5-6 times, although height-weight people are kind of lucky. When a person has a body mass index (BMI) of 25-30 and above, definitely, the person in question is certified as being obese.

Type 2 Diabetes

Type 2 diabetes is the most popular form of the disorder that covers the population with over 90 percent diagnosed persons. They are of two forms which are 1). insulin-dependent that genetically occurs when prediabetic, fasting blood glucose exceeds 125 mg/dL, or when your A1c level is greater than 6.5 and you're no longer capable of manufacturing adequate endogenous insulins. And 2). non insulin-independent that excels when the prediabetic, fasting blood glucose exceeds 125 mg/dL, or when your A1c level is greater than 6.5, but you're still manufacturing adequate endogenous insulin.

Most people with type 2 diabetes suffer from metabolism syndrome (an ideology that represents the process that causes insulin resistance and also the circumstance whereby the insulin is completely ineligible to produce beta cells. Metabolic syndrome is related to the following risk factors;

- Excessive weight gain and belly fat
- High blood sugar and high blood pressure
- Diet rejection most especially carbs
- Genetics inheritance

T2D's most dangerous, yet overlooked risk factor is weight gain which can be detected in almost 80% out of 90% of people with type 2 diabetes.

Being obese or overweight increases the chance of type 2 diabetes by 5-6 times, although height-weight people are kind of lucky. When a person has a body mass index (BMI) of 25-30 and above, definitely, the person in question is certified as being obese.

Obesity matriculates the progression of T2D, but doesn't determine it to be too serious because it can be manageable. Unlike T1D, you can live long for years if you eat a balanced, healthy diet and instructionally maintain the prescribed insulin availability whether through injections or pumps in T2D. Also, the risk of obesity can be tackled by following part of the *5 tricks* that concerns frequent day-to-day exercises.

Chapter 2

Mastering Diabetes Fundamentals

Worry less, you'll be fine. Initially, diabetes can be managed and indeed, cured. Various studies support the saying and oppositely, some studies and even some experts still never believe that a person can manage or recover from diabetes.

Are we even supposed to listen to the doubters? Does it mean a person with diabetes should ignore and wait for the chronic implications to dispense his/her life? The implications caused by diabetes alone are worth fearing but doesn't matter.

Different types of diabetes and sufferer metabolic state will determine the actual treatment protocol to be given. Both physical and medical alternatives are to work along this path. When managing diabetes, out of 100% available suggestions, 80% proclaim that by eating low-carb diet alone can cure the disease. Diabetes is complex. Most importantly, knowing the causes or factors worsening the disease can be the perfect way to fist on an accurate protocol to manage it.

What Exactly Causes Insulin Resistance?

I believe we all know that insulin resistance is the cause of diabetes as explained in each diabetes type above. The question is "what exactly is the root cause of insulin resistance in the body" and by doing so, clearance on protocol to use would be easy. Though, some attributes to lifestyle preference can indirectly impair insulin sensitivity, below is the most likely cause of insulin resistance.

Carbohydrates (carbs)— Without doubt, the most ardent source of insulin dysfunction is carbs in your meal. Carbs, in a normal circumstance, are the key source of energy. But for diabetes, this macronutrient has the greatest impact on a person's blood glucose, also known as blood sugar.

Carbohydrates in meals are classified into three hilarious types: starch, sugar, and fiber. Starches and sugars are the most problematic compound for a person suffering diabetes since the body converts them to glucose easily. Also with starches, usually before reaching our plates, starches are broken down through several pressures. This mechanism makes carbs from starch promptly/easily absorbed and converted into glucose by the body.

Insulin resistance does not occur immediately because of the carbohydrates absorption, but it happens when they are left spotted in the bloodstream with no response to exhale or lead them to possess energy. Insulin resistance starts to reflect when the carbohydrates instantly convert to sugar that stops your pancreas to produce an accurate amount of insulin for the muscle and liver to do their job.

Can Insulin Be Revived?

Story short, that's the goal. You're here to learn a long-term and feasible lifestyle that is capable of reducing and completely eliminating need for expenses on injective insulin while naturally, but effectively enhancing insulin sensitivity. The *5 Trick strategy* can help obtain a positive outcome and revitalize insulin sensitivity.

Key Basics For Reinstalling Insulin Resistance

When you're considering trying both scientifically proven, and natural remedies to help prevent insulin resistance or boost their energy to lower blood sugar, fisting on the following knowledge is necessary: 1). Nutrition value 2). Weight management

In today's world, doctors might have that great desire to make sure their patients are fine. But most especially, they are more prone to the use of surgical and pharmacological approaches in curiosity to disease of any kind. One thing I wish people could have known by now is that it is not every condition, most especially the chronic and severe ones that must be intercepted through surgical and pharmacological methods.

Food, yes I mean the food we all eat as either breakfast, lunch, and dinner is a very powerful healer in and of itself.

When we're talking about foods to maintain blood sugar, low-carb foods are your needs to cooperate.
When you eat any food that contains a surplus amount of carbohydrate energy irrespective of whether whole or processed, the carbohydrate

turns to glucose (sugar) as explained countlessly in the previous page.

Nutritional value is the right term for this and it's all about knowing foods that trigger both positive and negative effects in your body. There's a total difference between eating right, and eating healthy as a diabetes sufferer. A normal, healthy person is advised to keep all 6 classes of foods present before they can assume eating right. But for you, you don't need to eat right, you need to eat healthily. In that case, understanding the benefits of nutrition and criticizing a unique way to ensure eating healthy is important for repairing insulin sensitivity and entirely avoiding insulin resistance.

Weight Management

The second most customary and accessible approach geared for restoring and boosting insulin sensitivity is the need to make a distinctive routine for weight management. Diabetes alters a discrete master plan to cooperate with, and most especially in an appropriate way to stay away from certain facets. Organically, some diets may trigger you to lose weight and gain energy.

Other diets, or sometimes exactly the same that works for a friend, might decrease energy in you and cause weight gain. Obesity comes in.

The risk of obesity is currently molesting a large percentage of bloodlines, friends and families that are suffering type 2 diabetes across the globe. In fact, obesity is the major mainspring of high blood pressure and high cholesterol disorder. Several studies support this fact, and it's undoubtedly true.

Due to the fact that insulin is a hormone that helps you store fat, significant insulin spikes make you store more. You gain weight as a result of your liver's new ability to transform sugar into fats, which also increases your insulin sensitivity. However, sticking to an exercise regimen is indispensable for fat-burning, which in turn helps you lose weight and restore insulin resistance.

Chapter 3

Getting Started With Reversing Diabetes

Knowing Your Needs As A Diabetic

1. Eat healthy
2. Exercise steady
3. Try doing some meaningful and a bit stressful stuff to keep you active and less fatigued
4. Always stay hydrated
5. Stay consistent to the 5 *tricks* you'll discover soon in the next healdline.

6. Meet your doctor when feeling otherwise pressure and if possible, before trying any treatment for blood sugar
7. Get a journal to track your day to day A1c level, and blood sugar level.

Food Guide

1. Diet plans must be well balanced, but tailored to your choice.
2. Absorb moderate calories that can help you to shed or gain weight as needed while remaining close to your ideal/desirable body weight.
3. Completely stop the use of refined and starchy meals like maida, rava, white bread, potatoes, other tubers, processed foods, and meats.

4. Include plenty of veggies and one or two servings of fruits like oranges, papaya, mosambi, guava, or watermelon. Sweet taste fruits, such as Sitaphal (custard apple), chick, sweet bananas, grapes, and mangoes, must be avoided with no second choice.
5. Include foods strong in fiber (whole grains, legumes, and all green vegetables are accurate).
6. Aim for at least 20-35 g of fiber every day. Fibre aids in the reduction of postprandial blood glucose and cholesterol levels and eating plenty of them can assist.
7. Eat as many greens and vegetables as possible you can on a daily basis.
8. Stick to a low-glycemic-index diet to help keep blood sugar levels normal and on track.
9. Completely avoid saturated fats which are mostly present in butter, ghee, coconut oil, and palm oil.

10. Mustard oil, corn oil, sunflower oil, groundnut oil, rice bran oil, and ginger oil are all good choices because they contain less than 10% saturated fat and a 1:1 ratio of monounsaturated and polyunsaturated fats. Meanwhile, trans fats like margarine and dalda/vanaspati should be avoided.
11. Keep a food journal. Keep track of everything you consume in one day. You will be surprised at the volume and variety of food you consume and it will be easy to determine your glucose level.
12. If you're obese, you should limit your calorie consumption by reducing your carbohydrate and fat intake. Ensure that food is eaten not only at the appropriate time but also in the appropriate amount.
13. Include 4-6 small frequent meals rather than three large meals per day.

14. Make healthy choices when you go shopping, cooking, or eating out.
15. Always read labels and choose foods that are low in fat, salt, and sugar.
16. Drink sufficient, but moderate amounts of water everyday and don't let hunger depress you.
17. Salads should be included in lunch and dinner.
18. Avoid using table salt and limit your consumption of processed meals.

Trick 1

Starting A Healthy Low Gi Diet

The glycemic index (GI), is one of the best diets that is originally developed for diabetics to aid in blood sugar management. It is a wonderful trick of dieting that is feasible for both diabetics and those of us who simply want help planning meals and making healthier dietary choices. The GI is a measurement that determines how quickly our bodies convert carbs in our food into energy via glucose form. A score on the GI scale indicates how quickly this digestion occurs and how much it boosts glucose levels in the blood. Glucose is a norm for all other types of food and has a score of 100.

As elaborated above, every cell in our body needs glucose as its primary source of energy. When blood glucose levels begin to rise, the pancreas releases insulin, which encourages glucose uptake by cells and, as a result, returns blood sugar levels to a more controllable range.

Low-GI foods, such as lentils, beans, whole grains, nuts, and seeds, release energy slowly and help reduce sugar at its highs. If you typically consume a lot of high-GI foods which includes high amount of carbs concentrate like white bread, processed breakfast cereals, cakes, and biscuits, your body will have to work extremely hard to manage this and, if you are unable to use it as energy, the body will store it for later use. The later use is the starting point of insulin resistance or insulin insufficiency, diabetes follows.

The ratio of amylose to amylopectin, a kind of starch, determines whether a food has a low or high GI. Foods with a larger proportion of amylose, such as lentils, have lower GIs than foods with a higher proportion of amylopectin, such as potatoes.

When blood sugar (glucose) levels rise sharply, the pancreas releases more insulin to eradicate the excess glucose from the blood. Simultaneously, it slows the rate at which the body consumes fat as well. Focusing on low-GI carbohydrate items, on the other hand, promotes a continuous restriction to rise in blood glucose levels, which leads to a tiny and gradual rise in insulin. Small insulin surges keep you feeling complete and energized for hours after eating, and they may also encourage the body to burn fat.

How To Follow A Low GI Diet

To exact that you are adhering to a Low GI diet, understanding the Glycemic Index Foundation classification to the GI of food is important and it reads as follows:

- 70 or greater—High GI
- 56-69—Medium GI
- 55 or less—Low GI

Your goal is to maintain a no High, no Medium, but a healthy diet that is completely Low GI detected. Making it happen is not that complex, but can be so, due to unusual familiarity to new things. According to a recent study supporting the monitoring of GI foods, macronutrient content like protein and fat, fiber content, sugar and starches, ripeness and maturity of some food, processing, preparation, and cooking methods, the physical form of some food, anti-nutrients in some food, which are substances that can block the absorption of nutrients into the body altogether determines whether a food is Low GI or not.

Healthy Low GI foods

1. Protein rich foods. Lean meat, egg, and fish are some included examples
2. Unsweetened soy milk
3. Porridge made with pure steel-cut oats and water
4. Vegetables, including green peas, broccoli, and leafy greens
5. Dairy products, including milks and naturally-made yogurts
6. Legumes, beans, and pulses including lentils, chickpeas, and kidney beans

7. Low-sugar fruits. Apples, oranges, and blueberries are considerably included

Sample Breakfast

Semi-dried Tomato Omelette & Feta scramble
Prep time-5 minute|cook time-5 minute| serving-1
Ingredients:
- 2 eggs, firmly beaten
- 4 semi-dried tomatoes
- mixed salad leaves, to serve
- 25g feta cheese, crumbled
- 1 tsp olive oil

Instructions:
- Heat the 1 tsp oil in a small-sized frying pan, add the 2 eggs and cook, churning the eggs with a fork as they set.

- As the eggs are still slightly molten in the centre, scatter over the 4 semi-dried tomatoes and 25g feta cheese, then fold the omelette in half.
- Cook for an extra 1 min, more before sliding onto a plate. Serve alongside a mixed leaf salad to balance the GI level.

Sample Lunch

Vegetable Lentils with Egg Toast
Prep time-5 minute|cook time-10 minute| serving-2

Ingredients:
- ⅓ cup light brown sugar
- 2 cups old fashioned oats
- 1 ½ teaspoons cinnamon-ground
- 1 teaspoon baking powder

- ¼ teaspoon salt
- 1 ½ cups milk
- ½ cup unsweetened applesauce
- 2 tablespoons unsalted and firmly melted butter
- 1 large egg, beaten
- 1 teaspoon vanilla extract
- ⅓ cup raisins or dried cranberries

Instructions:
- Set up the oven's temperature you're using to 350°F. An 8x8-inch baking dish should be greased with nonstick cooking spray and left aside for some seconds or minutes.
- Combine the 2 cups of old fashioned oats, ⅓ cup light brown sugar, 1 ½ teaspoons ground cinnamon, baking powder, and ¼ teaspoon salt in a mixing basin.

- Combine 1 ½ cups milk, ½ cup unsweetened applesauce, 2 tablespoons unsalted and melted butter, 1 large egg, and 1 teaspoon vanilla extract in a medium bowl.
- To the oat mixture, add the milk mixture and stir thoroughly several times. Or add dried cranberries and raisins. Pour into the heated and sprayed pan to be ready to bake.
- Oatmeal will firm and instantly turn golden brown after 30 to 35 minutes of baking if you pour the mixture into the prepared pan.

Sample Dinner

Garlicky Shrimp & Broccoli

Prep time-5 minute|cook time-15 minute| serving-2

Ingredients:

- ½ pound deveined and peeled raw shrimp-(25-30 count)
- 3 medium cloves garlic, sliced, divided
- 2 cups broccoli florets-small ones
- 3 tablespoons extra-virgin olive oil, divide into 2 equal halves
- ½ cup diced red bell pepper
- ¼ teaspoon salt-divided
- ¼ teaspoon ground pepper, divided
- 1 teaspoons lemon juice, or more to taste

Ingredients:

- In a large pot, warm 1½ tablespoons of oil over medium heat. Cook for about a minute after adding half the garlic, or until it starts to color. Add the bell pepper, broccoli, and ⅛ teaspoons of salt and pepper. Until the veggies are soft, 3 to 5 minutes, cook with the lid on, stirring once or twice, and add 1 tablespoon water if the pot is too dry. Keep heated after transferring to a dish.

- Add the final tablespoon of oil to the pot and raise the heat to medium-high. About 1 minute later, add the remaining garlic and continue cooking until it starts to brown. Add the shrimp and the remaining ⅛ teaspoon of salt and pepper. Cook, stirring, for 3 to 5 minutes, or until the shrimp are barely cooked through. Add the lemon juice and the broccoli mixture back to the pot and stir to incorporate.

Trick 2

Intermittent Fasting For Weight Loss And Reestablishing Insulin Sensitivity

Intermittent fasting has become popular in recent years as an effective, and perhaps best weight loss method. When on intermittent fasting, you only eat for a specific window of time. Fasting for a set number of hours per day or eating only one meal a few times per week can assist your body in burning fat. According to several studies and research, intermittent fasting can reduce your risk of diabetes and heart disease, with clear proof to back it up.

Type 2 diabetes is not always a chronic, life-long illness. Diabetes remission is feasible if you lose weight through dietary and activity changes. Intermittent fasting is more of shading off excess weight with a "no too much eating" pattern which would help boost insulin sensitivity and decrease blood sugar. In the "no too much eating" pattern, intermittent fasting triggers the pancreas to produce and release sufficient glucagon, the hormone in charge of preventing glucose from dropping too low.

Based on the 5 trick strategy, intermittent fasting is the second most powerful trick after a low GI diet. The basic purpose of intermittent fasting for weight loss is to lower insulin levels so that your body burns stored fat (rather than sugar) for energy.

Since it can help relieve type 2 diabetes, the question now is, how do you get started? Not a big deal. All you need to know to get started is what to do and how to do it in intermittent fasting, of which you will find in the next paragraph.

Everything You Need To Know Before Getting Started With This Trick

Consult your diabetic team to see if the pattern is right for you. Any adjustments to your medication schedule should be made in accordance with their recommendations. The goal is to maintain a healthy blood glucose level, whereas in a safe manner.

Check your blood glucose levels frequently.

If you experience hypoglycemic symptoms, you should break your fast right away. Use your action plan, such as taking glucose pills followed by a snack. Before resuming the fast, consult with your doctor.

If you have type 1 diabetes, keep an eye out for indicators of hyperglycemia during fasting. These symptoms include weariness, severe thirst, and frequent urination. If you have these symptoms or your blood sugar level remains high, contact your healthcare professional straight away.

How To Do It

- Avoid dehydration by drinking enough fluids during the fast. Avoid sugary beverages. Instead, during the fast, drink adequate water.

- In order to acquire enough fiber, protein, vitamins, and minerals, eat meals from all food categories/groups.
- During the non-fasting periods, avoid overeating.
- Eat items that will keep you full and your blood sugar stable during the fast. Lean protein, beans, nuts, fruits, veggies, and fresh salads are all good examples you could adhere to.
- Eat slower-absorbing foods, such as those with a lower glycemic index, just before fasting. They are frequently heavy in fiber or protein and are slow to digest.
- Limit the amount or portion of greasy and sugary foods when you break the fast. Instead of frying, consider grilling or baking stuff.

Trick 3

Exercising To Regain Insulin Sensitivity

It is well known that acute, short-term exercise greatly increases insulin sensitivity. Moderate-intensity exercise can increase glucose absorption by 40% or more in a single workout session. With post-exercise assessments done between 12 and 48 hours following the last session, a number of early studies demonstrated significant increases in glucose tolerance and insulin sensitivity in response to exercise training.

This is reinforced by the fact that among trained individuals, stopping exercise is associated with a significant and rapid drop in insulin sensitivity. In addition, exercise promotes weight loss, which reverses the insulin resistance that is a hallmark of obesity. Therefore, if daily exercise was also accompanied by less body fat, the positive effect on insulin resistance would be amplified. It is the third successful treatment approach for reducing insulin resistance and, more significantly, improving overall quality of life and well-being. In addition, modest exercise lowers the morbidity and mortality linked to cardiovascular disease and diabetes as well.

Exercise routines can help persons like you with diabetes who are insulin resistant get your condition under control. Regular exercise helps to reduce body fat, which increases cellular insulin sensitivity since extra adiposity around the waist contributes to insulin resistance. Due to an increase in the amount of GLUT4 (Glucose Transporter type 4) in plasma membranes and T-tubules, glucose absorption is maintained at a higher level for up to 120 minutes following physical activity. At least 16 hours after exercising, insulin sensitivity increases. Both persons with type 2 diabetes and healthy people have this noticed in them. Physical exercise may also improve lipid metabolism and control hepatic glucose output, both of which are crucial in type 2 diabetes.

Why Do You Need To Exercise?

There is so much reason why you should exercise as long as diabetes is concerned. Both long term and should term exercise activities can boost insulin sensitivity and some other potential benefits such as:

- Exercise of any kind, whether it be aerobic, resistance, or a combination of the two (combined training), can lower HbA1c levels in diabetics.
- In inactive older people with abdominal obesity who might be at risk for diabetes, resistance training and aerobic exercise can both help to reduce insulin resistance. Compared to their inactive counterparts, people with diabetes who exercise three to four hours a week will reduce their risk of dying from heart disease
- Women with diabetes who engage in moderate (including walking) or strenuous exercise for at least four hours per week have a 40% possibility of a decreased chance of getting heart

disease than those who does not exercise. Even after confounding variables like BMI, smoking, and other heart disease risk factors were taken into account by the researchers, these advantages persisted.

Suitable Exercise For Diabetics

Walking—Many people prefer walking since it is a low-impact activity that almost every person does everyday. Increasing your step count as a diabetes sufferer will lower your cholesterol, blood pressure, and glucose levels. You might see it as too common, but the effectiveness is mind-blowing. The American Diabetes Association's (ADA) recommendation for daily cardiovascular activity is 30 minutes of brisk walking, or roughly 100 steps per minute. You might increase the intensity of your walking exercises when you include activities like stair climbing. Nevertheless, 100 steps per minute or more would go a long way.

Running—You can progress from brisk walking to parade running with the right training and the endorsement of your physical doctor. A daily 50-100 metre run everyday will help burn fat, while on the process, the risk of high blood pressure, high blood sugar, and excessive cholesterol will reduce

Cycling—There is a good reason why stationary bikes are so well-liked. The health of your heart and lungs as well as your balance and posture can all be enhanced after some specific regular riding. But to begin, you do not need a pricey workout bike. Grab an old bike and head outside, or check out the stationary bikes at your neighbourhood gym, and stroll down the street.

Dancing—Your exercise program may become more enjoyable if you incorporate dance. Dancing is a heart-healthy activity that also helps with blood sugar control and fitness. According to one study, those with T2D who took part in dance classes were more likely to stick to a routine than those who followed a different fitness regimen. You'll lose weight, and as well be happy like never before especially when done with friends.

Water aerobics—There are many benefits to exercising in the water or pool. Swimming and other water exercises are gentle on the joints and may lower blood sugar levels. Additionally, they might improve heart health, overall strength, and fitness in any T2D patient including you if you're one.

High intensity interval training—HIIT, an abbreviation for high intensity interval training, involves alternating between brief bursts of high-intensity exercise and prolonged bouts of lower-intensity motion. It can be added to a variety of workouts, including cycling and running. HIIT, when done together with running and cycling would help your Type 2 diabetes and lower your fasting blood sugar.

Weight training—Weights or other heavy equipment are used in this type of strength training to increase or maintain muscular mass and strength. This will help you burn fats and would improve your glucose tolerance and insulin sensitivity.

Yoga—Yoga combines breathing, meditation, and gentle movement of the body that improves balance, flexibility, and strength. If you're an elderly T2D patient who may be more at risk of falling, trying different types of yoga poses would help you retain balance, and at the same, you'll be able to control your cholesterol and blood sugar levels with the practice.

5 Best Quick Exercise to keep you active

Crunch back—Lie on your back, your feet flat on the floor, and your knees bent. Lock your hands behind your head. Draw your one shoulder blade closer to the meet the other and your elbows back. The elbows should focus sideways and remain in place throughout the exercise. Curdle your abs and twine your shoulders and upper back off the floor.

Bend down slowly. Do not lift ur back off the floor until you're done.

Flat Plank—With your palms down and toes tucked in, lie face-down with your elbows directly beneath your shoulders. Lift your body and thighs off the ground while contracting your back, glutes, and abs from this beginning position. Toes and forearms will support you. Spend at least five seconds in this position. Slowly descend to the starting posture while maintaining a flat straight back.

Lower Body Squat—Place your feet shoulder-width apart and maintain a standing position. As though you were sitting in a chair, lower yourself by bending your knees. Your knees should not protrude past your toes, and your thighs should be parallel to the ground. As you get back up, lean slightly forward.

Hamstring Curl—Take hold of a chair's back. Bring your left foot's heel toward your butt while bending your knee. Your right leg needs to be slightly bent as well. Put your left foot back on the ground. Repeat with the right leg after completing 8–12 reps. If you want to make this exercise more challenging, see if wearing ankle weights is safe for you and give it a try.

Lower Body Lunges—Step your right leg back while keeping it from touching the floor as you stand with your legs shoulder-width apart. Your left thigh ought to be almost parallel to the ground. Returning the right leg to a neutral position, press down on the left heel. Do 8–12 repetitions on one side, then switch by stepping back with your left leg. Hold a dumbbell in each hand to make the lunges harder if possible.

Trick 4

Knowing your pros and cons as a diabetic

The type of diabetes you suffer today is a repercussion of not knowing what to do. Maybe, or even doing things you feel are right to do, whereas they're not. According to an adage, the earlier you approach, the better it becomes. Anyway, if you've already been diagnosed with any form of diabetes, especially T2D, below is a breakdown of the do's and don't you should stick to.

10 Foods To Completely Avoid

---

1. Chocolates & desserts
2. High sugar fruits like grapes, chikoo, and custard apple
3. Maida products like white bread, pasta
4. Rice and biryanis
5. Dried fruits
6. Packaged foods like chips, cookies, and other fierce fried munchies
7. Fried foods like samosas, fries, pakodas
8. Potatoes and tubers
9. Packaged and sugar-added beverages
10. Some milk products like creamy milk and or cheese

10 Modification To Make Instead

1. Chocolates and desserts can be substituted with sugar-free and fat-free options since they are unavoidable.

2. Fruits like bananas, grapes, chikoo, & custard apples should be completely avoided with no second thought. Opt for healthier options like citrus fruits, berries, papaya, pomegranate and more less-ripped and less-sugar fruits.

3. Maida products like white bread, pasta should be avoided as well and swapped for multigrain healthy bread and pure Atta pasta which are much lower in calories and very similar in taste.

4. Rice and biryanis should go with khichdi, or brown rice as they both taste alike while lower in carb.

5. Dried fruits – Fruits are dried but retain the sugar content, so it is better to eat the permitted

and fresh variety of fruits just to ensure eating what you want in a healthy manner.

6. Packaged foods like chips, cookies, and other munchies- there is no second choice alternative to such foods. Sorry to say, they are a no-go area, avoid them.

7. Fried foods like samosas, fries, pakodas- these staple Indian tea-time snacks are bombs which can explode anytime to cause inflammation and so forth. Opt for salad vegetables or fruits and substitute milky tea with green tea instead.

8. Try sweet potatoes instead of the popular potato curry recipes.

9. Packaged and sugar-added beverages- Green tea or fresh juice are good options to swap them.

10. Some milk products like creamy milk, cheese- these have healthy options like fat-free or toned milk, paneer, curds to go with.

Best Food List Diagram For Diabetes

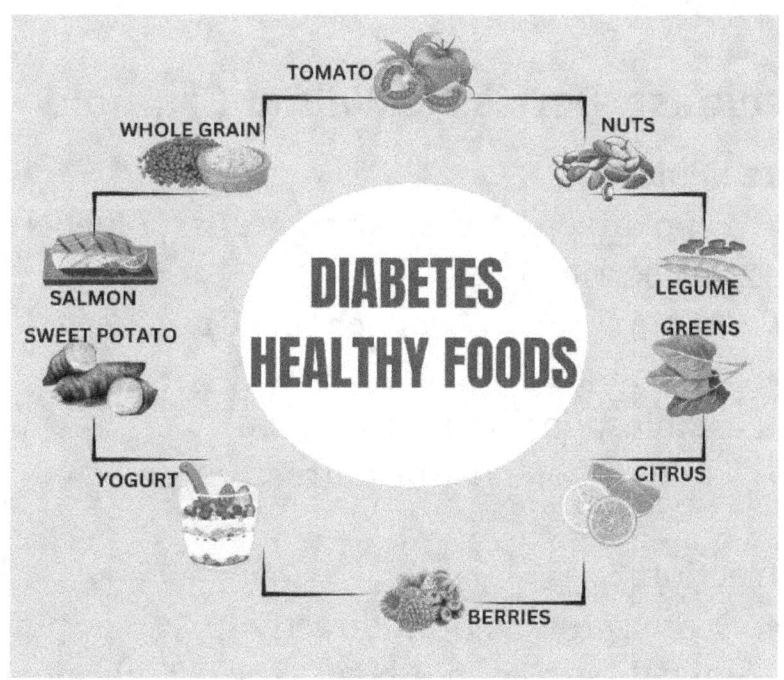

Meal Plan & Recipes

Day 1

Breakfast: Berries & Walnut Crumble

Ingredients:
- 1 cup mixed berries (strawberries, blueberries, raspberries.)
- ¼ cup walnuts (well-chopped)
- ¼ cup oats
- 2 tablespoon honey (optional)
- 1 tablespoon healthy butter

Instructions:
- Switch the oven on directly to 375°F, put the mixed berries in a bowl with 1 tablespoon of

honey or maple syrup (if using), and then mix properly.

- Combine the oats, chopped walnuts, and remaining honey or maple syrup (if using) in a separate bowl.
- Set a little skillet over medium heat and melt the butter.
- The combination of oats and walnuts should be added to the skillet and cooked for approximately 3 to 5 minutes, stirring regularly, until completely toasted.
- Spread the mixed berries in a baking dish, then sprinkle the oat and walnut mixture on top.
- Bake in the preheated oven for approximately 15 to 20 minutes, or until the topping is golden brown.
- Serve and enjoy.

Lunch: Red Pepper Dip serrved With Whole Grain Vegetables

Ingredients:
- 2 red bell peppers (well-roasted and peeled)
- ½ cup low-fat Greek yogurt
- 1 tablespoon lemon juice
- 1 clove garlic
- Salt to taste
- Pepper to taste

Instructions:
- The roasted red peppers should be smoothed out in a food processor.
- Blend in the Greek yogurt, lemon juice, and garlic until thoroughly blended.
- Add pepper alongside with salt to your desired taste.
- Serve and enjoy as a dip with whole-grain crackers or vegetables.

Dinner: Mussel and Crab Fry

Ingredients:

- 1 tablespoon olive oil
- 1 small onion
- 1½ cloves garlic
- ½ teaspoon chilli flakes (optional)
- Salt to taste
- 1 pound cleaned & debearded mussels
- 6 ounces crabmeat
- Pepper to taste
- 1 teaspoon paprika

Instructions:

- In a small-sized skillet over medium-high heat, warm the olive oil. The onion and garlic should be added and simmered until tender.

- The mussels should be added to the skillet and cooked until they begin to open broadly.
- Crabmeat, paprika, and chili flakes (if wanted) should all be stirred in. Cook for a further and approximately 2 to 3 minutes.
- To taste, Sprinkle the salt and pepper as desired on the food. Serve warm.

Day 2

Breakfast: Ham & Cheddar Omelette

Ingredients:
- 2 eggs
- pepper to taste
- 2 slices of ham (well-diced)
- ¼ cup cheddar cheese (well-shredded)
- 1 tablespoon healthy butter
- Spicy unsalted spices

Instructions:
- Begin by whisking the eggs together in a sizeable bowl, add the salt and pepper to it.
- Melt the healthy butter or heat oil in a non-stick pan over a medium-high temperature.
- Cook the ham in diced form for approximately one to two minutes, or until it turns faintly browned.
- Over the ham, pour the whisked eggs, and simmer for approximately two to three minutes.
- Then, fold the omelet in half while spreading the cheddar cheese shreds on top of the eggs.
- Cook the eggs for an additional 1−2 minutes, or until they are fully cooked and the cheese has properly melted.

Lunch: Lentil Herbs Salad

Ingredients:
- 1 cup lentils (cooked)
- ¼ cup chopped parsley
- ¼ chopped mint
- ¼ chopped cilantro
- Spicy unsalted spices
- Pepper to taste
- ¼ cup diced red onion
- ¼ cup diced cucumber
- 1 tbsp lemon juice
- 1 tbsp olive oil

Instructions:
- In a big-sized bowl, mix all herbs and ingredients together, and gently toss them to coat.
- If required, taste and adjust the seasoning.
- Serve and enjoy.

Dinner: Peach Salmon

Ingredients:
- 1½ salmon fillets
- Salt and pepper to taste
- Fresh herbs (like dill or basil) for garnish (optional)
- 1½ peaches
- 1 tablespoon olive oil
- ½ tablespoon lemon juice

Instructions:
- Set the oven's temperature to 400°F (200°C).
- The salmon fillets should be placed on a baking pan covered with parchment paper.
- Over the salmon, drizzle some lemon juice and olive oil. Add salt and pepper (as desired).

- Place the salmon fillets on a plate and top with the peach slices.
- When the salmon is cooked through and flakes easily with a fork, bake in the preheated oven for a maximum of 12 to 15 minutes.
- If preferred, garnish and enjoy with the fresh herbs before serving.

Day 3

Breakfast: Bread and Egg White with Oat

Ingredients:
- 1 slice of whole wheat bread
- 1 egg
- ¼ cup rolled oats
- Salt to taste
- Pepper to taste
- 1 tsp olive oil

Instructions:
- Over medium heat, gently preheat a nonstick skillet.
- Beat the egg in a bowl and season with salt and pepper to taste.
- Dip each slice of bread in the egg mixture, and be careful to cover both sides.
- Gently push down to help the rolled oats adhere as you roll the bread in them.
- Grease the heated skillet with the olive oil, then add the coated bread inside.
- Cook for approximately 2 to 3 minutes on each side or until well-cooked and browned.

Lunch: Salsa Salmon Salad

Ingredients:
- 1 salmon (4-6 ounces) fillet

- 1½ cups mixed salad greens
- ½ cup cherry tomatoes, halved
- ¼ cup diced cucumber
- ½ cup diced red onion
- 1½ tablespoons salsa (choose a sugar-free variety)
- 1 tablespoon extra-virgin olive oil
- 1 tablespoon freshly squeezed lemon juice
- Salt to taste
- Pepper to taste

Instructions:
- Set the oven's temperature to 400°F (200°C). On a baking sheet covered with parchment paper, put the salmon fillet, and add salt and pepper to taste.
- The salmon should be baked for 12 to 15 minutes, or until it flakes easily with a fork chunk.

- Combine and mix the salad greens, cherry tomatoes, cucumber, and red onion in a big bowl.
- To create the dressing, combine the salsa, olive oil, lemon juice, salt, and pepper in a small different bowl.
- Cook, then flake the salmon into small pieces and stir it into the salad dressing.
- Over the salad, drizzle the dressing, and toss continuously to mix.
- Serve the salmon salad with the salsa and enjoy it right away.

Dinner: Quinoa Lime Beans Salad

Ingredients:
- 1 cup quinoa (cooked)
- ½ red onion, chopped
- ¼ cup chopped fresh cilantro

- 1½ tablespoons lime juice
- 1 can black beans (drained and rinsed)
- 1 cup cherry tomatoes, halved
- 2 tablespoons olive oil
- Salt to taste
- Pepper to taste

Instructions:
- Combine and whisk together the cooked quinoa, black beans, cherry tomatoes, red onion, and cilantro in a medium-sized bowl.
- Mix the lime juice, olive oil, salt, and pepper in a separate small bowl.
- Toss in the arranged quinoa salad with the mixed dressing to coat.
- Keep chilled until you're ready to serve.

Trick 5

Admiring Medical Necessity For Checkups

Although the 4 explained tricks can eliminate insulin resistance, it's important to know whether what you've been doing is really improving your blood sugar, which is why the need for medical checkup whether weekly or daily is important.

Just as adviced in the previous chapter, getting a Medically approved tracking journal for yourself, one of a kind that includes pages for monitoring your AIC level and carb intake can help. Meet your medical doctor for it. It's the best way to thrive on your journey to mastering diabetes with happiness.

Diabetes is a disorder. Thrive in it with the 5 tricks strategy. Hopefully, you'll conquer it!